YOUR KNOWLEDGE HAS VALUE

- We will publish your bachelor's and master's thesis, essays and papers

- Your own eBook and book - sold worldwide in all relevant shops

- Earn money with each sale

Upload your text at www.GRIN.com
and publish for free

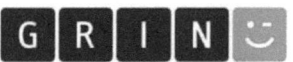

Bibliographic information published by the German National Library:

The German National Library lists this publication in the National Bibliography; detailed bibliographic data are available on the Internet at http://dnb.dnb.de .

Imprint:

Copyright © 2018 GRIN Verlag
Print and binding: Books on Demand GmbH, Norderstedt Germany
ISBN: 9783668676091

This book at GRIN:

https://www.grin.com/document/418400

Patrick Kimuyu

Leadership as an Integral Element in Healthcare

GRIN Verlag

GRIN - Your knowledge has value

Since its foundation in 1998, GRIN has specialized in publishing academic texts by students, college teachers and other academics as e-book and printed book. The website www.grin.com is an ideal platform for presenting term papers, final papers, scientific essays, dissertations and specialist books.

Visit us on the internet:

http://www.grin.com/

http://www.facebook.com/grincom

http://www.twitter.com/grin_com

Leadership as an Integral Element in Healthcare

Name: Patrick Kimuyu

Contents

Introduction

Leadership seems to have become a powerful tool in organizational management. This is attributable to the notion that leaders, rather than managers have significant influences in legitimate organizations. According to Bertocci (2009), one of the key reasons why leadership has become an integral element in recent years is because of the evolving nature of the business world which has become more competitive, more global and more volatile. It is also apparent that organizations are increasingly becoming technologically complex; thus, demanding a high level of expert power. Given the evolving nature of today's workplace environment and dynamics in the business world, it is explicit that leadership enhances organizational effectiveness through improving production, flexibility, competitiveness, quality, efficiency, satisfaction, and development. This is consistent with the opinion held by social scientists and organizational management experts who believe that effective leadership results into a level of order and consistency to the profitability, as well as quality of products and services. On the other hand, Lunenburg (2012) observes that a true leader promotes organizational effectiveness through influencing others and modifying their behavior. In retrospect, leadership has not been a complex task, but the evolving workplace environment due to changes in organizational structure and design are increasingly driving evolution in leadership. In order to cope with the current organizational change, it is believed that effective leadership is essential for organizational survival. Therefore, this research paper provides a focused discussion on leadership, qualities of a leader, today's workforce leadership challenges, and outcomes of good/bad leadership in a healthcare organization.

What Is Leadership?

From a retrospective point of view, it is apparent that different scholars view leadership from different perspectives. Therefore, the definition of leadership can be obtained from a focused reflection on these definitions.

First, the earliest definition of leadership is found in Stogdill's publication, 'Handbook of Leadership' which has emerged as one of the most authoritative sources of leadership theory. In his book, Stogdill (1974) seeks to define leadership based on the actions of a leader within a group. He describes a leader as an agent of change, an individual whose acts have more effects on other individuals more than the way other individuals' acts affect him. As such, Stogdill defines leadership as "an interaction between members or a group" (p. 43). He goes further to describe how leadership occurs. According to Stogdill (1974) leadership is manifested when a member in a group assumes the roles of modifying the competencies or motivation of other members in the group. As such, he somehow perceives leadership as the aspect of using influence. It is also suggestive that leadership can be manifested in interpersonal relationships. Overall, this definition seems to put emphasis the ability of being a change agent; that explicit ability to influence a follower's performance, or behavior.

Second, George and Gareth (2005) provide a relatively broad definition of leadership. They define leadership as one member's exercise of influence over other members of a group or organization with the aim of guiding the group towards achieving its goals. In this perspective, a leader is the group member who exerts this form of influence within an organization or group. Based on their perspective, these social scientists provide a distinction between informal and formal leaders. They describe an informal leader as one who exercises influence over followers through the use of their skills, friendship, or talent, but lacks formal authority. In contrast, they describe a formal leader as one who holds a virtual position within an organization, and has authority.

Third, Gibson, Ivancevich and Donnelly (2000) propose an interesting definition of leadership. They view leadership as a process through which one member of a group influences other members of the group to achieve desired goals without coercive influence. Based on this perspective, these scholars define leadership as "an attempt to use non coercive influence to motivate individuals to accomplish some goal" (p. 272).

Finally, Bertocci (2009) summarizes these definitions of leadership and comes up with what he refers to as the working definition of leadership. He defines leadership as the aspect of combining personality traits which are possessed by an individual which enables that individual to exert influence on others through inspiration to accomplish goals which would not be achieved without the leader's motivation.

To summarize, it is explicit from these definitions that influence underpins leadership. A leader emerges as an individual who exhibits the qualities of a change agent; the ability to influence and modify other people's behavior, as well as performance. It is also apparent that these definitions emphasize on the achievement of the group's or organization's set goals. In this context, a leader is projected as an individual who understands the vision and mission of an organization. He is someone who can describe the past and the current state of an organization, as well as predict where the organization is heading to in the future. This way, they understand the path towards the accomplishment of the organizational goals and objectives. As such, he guides his followers through that path to realize the desired outcomes. Therefore, a leader's effectiveness in an organization can be measured depending on the accomplishment of the desired goals (Gibson, Ivancevich & Donnelly, 2000).

However, Gibson, Ivancevich and Donnelly (2000) observe that the effectiveness of a leader cannot be measured, accurately due to a number of reasons. First, there is an increasing tendency in organizations through which the selection of leaders is based on the similarity with previous leaders, especially on experiences, background and qualifications. As such, individuals who posses valuable leadership characteristics, but shares little similarity with previous leaders is not chosen to lead. This mode of selecting leaders within an organization has been found to enhance self-selection bias in which existing leader choose those whom they share similarities to succeed them. The second reason why measuring leadership effectiveness is because leaders do not have the capability of controlling all the factors relating to a given situation. They can only control, or modify behaviors and performance of their followers. For instance, a leader may lack the capability to control external factors which are outside their control such as policies, environmental factors and dynamics in the labor market. Given the fact that these factors influence leadership effectiveness, and yet they are outside leaders' control, it is implicit that measuring the effectiveness of leadership with precision is quite difficult. Finally, most leaders lack unilateral control over resources so they depend on the support of others to accomplish their leadership goals. For instance, some leaders require review, or approval of their decisions by other senior members within an organizational structure. At some circumstance, their decisions go through modifications, or even get rejected at the highest levels. This means that a leader's ability to drive his group towards a desired goal may be challenged by influence by other decision-makers; making it difficult to measure leadership effectiveness.

Differences between Leaders and Managers

From a critical perspective, leaders and leadership are intertwined. It is not possible to discuss one and leave the other. However, leaders are quite different from managers. As such, it is worth discussing the core functional differences that put leaders and managers on two diverse paths.

George and Gareth (2005) attempt to highlight the functional differences between leaders and managers based on the effectiveness is measured. They posit that accomplishment of goals serves as a measure of a leader's effectiveness. In contrast, a manager's effectiveness can simply be measured through the evaluation the profit margins. Another functional difference that sets leaders and managers in different functional paths is the way they exert their influence on their followers. A leader achieves an attractive outcome only if his followers accept his directives. As such, followers are at liberty to follow the leader or not. On the management side, managers are placed over the followers, or rather employees under the hierarchical organizational structure. In this scenario, employees are subject to the manager's directives and orders.

Another key difference between leaders and managers is that leaders focus on the organizational vision, change, big picture issues, and the future (Pierce & Robinson, 2007). In contrast, managers are concerned with complexity in personnel issues, control of input and output, staffing, and organization design (Kotter, 1992).

Bertocci (2009) explains the difference between leaders and managers from the perspective of how accomplish or cope with their primary responsibilities and functions. On the side of leadership, leaders cope with complexity at the workplace through developing a vision that addresses the change. As such, the vision guides the team towards accomplishing organizational goals while overcoming complexity challenges. To achieve this, leaders design a

5

strategy, communicate it to their followers and empower them to implement the strategy. This way, the strategy enhances the accomplishment of the task, bringing desirable outcomes. In contrast, managers cop with complexity through different means. They plan, set goals, develop a budget, and allocate resources, especially through staffing to accomplish their plans. Additionally, they monitor employees' adherence to the plan to ensure the accomplishment of the intended goals.

Finally, Kozak (1998) posits that both leadership and management are required for the success on any organization. Therefore, he outlines an array of characteristics that illustrate functional differences between leaders and managers. One of the key differences between leaders and managers is their orientation within an organization; leaders are usually results and goal-oriented, whereas managers are action and task-oriented. Another key difference as highlighted by Kozak (1998) is that leaders effective long-term planners, whereas managers are efficient short-term planners. He further states that leaders carry on their responsibilities through inspiring or empowering their followers, unlike it the case for managers who execute their responsibilities through directing their employees on what to do. Moreover, it is reported that leaders attract talents, whereas managers recruit talents.

Overall, it is explicit that there are significant differences between leadership and management. In this context, the key differences are associated from the way leaders and managers go about their functions within organizations, but not necessarily from themselves. However, their followers may not see the differences between leadership and management; instead, they judge their seniors based on their levels of friendliness.

Leadership Theories

Leadership can also be described through the use of leadership theories which explain the process of leadership. Over the past decades, a number of leadership theories have been proposed; thus, shaping the way leadership occurs within organizations. This implies that some leadership models are better than others. As such, organizational success in terms of effectiveness and productivity relies on the type of leadership model it adopts.

In this context, a brief discussion of the major assumptions and principles that underlie the main leadership theories explains the strength and weaknesses of a given theory. George and Gareth (2005) reviewed the key assumptions of leadership theories and prepared a concise summary. To start with, trait theory holds that possess identifiable personality characteristics which underpins their leadership capabilities. On the other hand, behavioral theory posits that leaders can be distinguished on the basis of specific behaviors. In contrast, the genetic theory of leadership holds that leadership traits are inheritable. It implies that successful leaders acquire leadership traits from their parents. As such, this theory is relatively the opposite of the Fiedler's contingency theory that holds that the effectiveness of leaders is determined by situations. It emphasizes that leaders tend to be task-oriented. Finally, path-goal theory and transformational theory are based on the influence of leaders on their followers. Transformational theory holds that leaders can use charisma to enhance their followers' productivity. Similarly, the path-goal theory posits that leaders can use motivational approaches to influence the performance of their followers towards the achievement of desired goals.

What Are Good/Bad Characteristics Of A Leader?

From a critical perspective, it is apparent that leaders can never be the same. They may achieve the same degree of leadership effectiveness, but there still exists significant differences, especially based on their leadership characteristics which range from personal traits to functional characteristics. On the same note, leaders do not produce similar influences on their followers, as well as organizational effectiveness. This is why some leaders are considered as good, whereas other are perceived as bad. Therefore, it is logical to deduce the key characteristics of good leaders and bad leaders based on the main leadership theories.

In practice, a good leader is celebrated by all stakeholders in the community, or within an organization (Gibson, Ivancevich & Donnelly, 2000). This aspect is attributable to the fact that good leadership generates numerous benefits to all parties. For instance, followers pay royalty to good leaders due to their satisfaction. This, in turn, enhances the attainment of organizational goals; thus, increasing the effectiveness, productivity and competitiveness of an organization.

Characteristics of a Good Leader

Charisma

One of the desirable characteristics of a good leader is charisma as it is put forward through the transformational leadership theory. It is reported that charisma underpins the effectiveness of leaders. It eases the task of getting followers heed to their leaders' call through positive influence. Through the use of charisma, a leader is able to align his followers' efforts towards achieving the vision of an organization. In addition, charisma serves as a useful tool for instilling ac sense of value, pride and respect amongst the followers (Gibson, Ivancevich & Donnelly 2000). According to the precepts of transformational leadership theory, a charismatic leader is able to increase followers' awareness of the significance of good performance, as well as the importance of their duties. They are also able to make the followers aware of the importance of their personal growth, accomplishment and development.

Finally, Bertocci (2009) observes that charisma serves as a reliable tool in solving crises at the workplace. He posits that a crisis-based charismatic leader is able to manage crisis where existing procedures, resources and knowledge are inadequate to solve the situation. This type of a leader can empower his followers to execute the required actions to solve the situation in relatively non-traditional actions. Gibson, Ivancevich & Donnelly (2000) proposes Steve Jobs, the cofounder of Apple Company as a charismatic leader.

Attentive

A good leader demonstrates a sense of attention to the needs of others. As such, he is able to assign meaningful strategies which promote personal and professional growth of his followers (Gibson, Ivancevich & Donnelly 2000). Second, a leader who is attentive to the needs of his followers is able to address external issues that may impair a follower's productivity. Third, an attentive leader is able to communicate efficiently with his followers. They are able to pass over ideas related to the vision to their followers and this enhances the accomplishment of goals. It is also worth noting that being attentive to followers creates an avenue for addressing the emerging concerns of followers leading to work satisfaction.

Motivational

Ability to motivate others to achieve a certain goal has an exceptional importance in leadership. According to the path-goal theory, a leader's behavior is usually motivational in nature. This is consistent with the principle definition of leadership which emphasize on the leader's ability to inspire his followers to achieve desired goals. A motivational leader provides clarity of direction, guidance and rewards his followers for effective performance (Gibson, Ivancevich & Donnelly 2000).

Ambitious

From a critical perspective, staying focused on achieving desired goals is the most essential requirement of success in all undertakings, either within organizational settings, or in daily life engagements. This implies that a successful leader can be identified based on the level of ambition .in this context, leader's degree of ambition can be evaluated using three leadership characteristics. Kirkpatrick and Locke (1991) observe that energy, tenacity and initiative as the key features of effective leadership. An ambitious leader channels his energy on accomplishing their goals no matter how intense or complex they may proof to be. On the other hand, an ambitious leader demonstrates tenacity; the ability to stay in power in the course of accomplishing complex tasks, or overcoming organizational challenges. Finally, ambition is demonstrated by the leader's initiative. This involves initiating any available opportunity to enhance the accomplishment of projects, as well as taking appropriate actions to address any underlying challenges. As such, an ambitious leader exhibits the quality of being proactive.

Self-confidence

A good leader remains bold at all situations. This is the ability of self-confidence; that inner assurance of competence within an individual. In practice, self-confidence forms an integral element that enables leaders to exert influence on their followers. A self-confident leader is able to motivate his followers endure difficult situations and remain resilient until appreciable outcomes are achieved (George & Gareth 2005).

Integrity and Honesty

Honesty defines an individual's nobility. These are some of the personality traits which are identified under the trait theory of leadership. Therefore, leadership which is founded on ethics demands integrity and honesty from leaders. This enables leaders to win their followers' trust and confidence (George & Gareth 2005).

Characteristics of a Bad Leader

Concisely, the lack of the characteristics which define a good leader as discussed above implies bad leadership. Some of the main characteristics of a bad leader include self-centeredness, poor communication, lack of personal accountability, poor decision-making ability, domineering, manipulative, arrogant, and inconsiderate.

According to Cohn and Moran (2011), a bad leader demonstrates lack of integrity, empathy, emotional intelligence, and passion. They consider these characteristics to be the essential requirements of good leadership. On the other hand Pandey (2014) identifies self-centeredness and the 'know-it-all' attitude as some of the key characteristics of a bad leader. They also note that a bad leader cannot lead by example. In other words, he lacks the ability to inspire his followers, especially through demonstrating the capability to perform what he delegates to his followers.

What Are Problems Leaders Face In Today's Workforce?

From a critical perspective, it is explicit that the society changes and develops at a rapid pace. As change is occurs in the society, change of similar magnitude is taking place at the workplace. In general, the 21st century workplace environment reflects significant differences from the earlier environment. All this has come with new leadership and managerial challenges. Evidence indicates that leaders are facing numerous challenges in today's workforce. Some of the major challenges that are faced by the 21st century leader in the workforce include demographic shifts, technological advancement, globalization, and work-life balance.

Demographic shift

In principle, it is apparent that the 21st century organization requires leaders to exhibit a significant shift in how they lead today's employee. Unlike it was in the past century, the era of the Baby Boomers, the millennials demonstrate an existence of a demographic shift at the workplace. Generation Y is poised to introduce a significant culture change in today's workplace, and this poses a threat to traditional leadership that was effective for generation X. However, it is worth noting that this demographic shift present challenges and opportunities for all organizations. This implies that any organization that intents to harness the benefits of this demographic shift must overcome the accompanying challenges. In practice, any demographic change within an organization demands change in leadership, in order to align changes in the workforce with organizational effectiveness.

To understand the need for changes in the way leaders lead and adopt new leadership strategies, it is worth shading some light on the situation in past and the present. If today's leaders are to steer success in today's organizations, they need to monitor dynamics in the economic climate. Overall, demographic shift has had an irrevocable impact on the business landscape. For instance, it was possible to predict an organization's future success by evaluating its past performance. This is contrary to the situation today where success is predicted by the level of evolution. It has become a requirement that organizations must exhibit continued evolution, in order to achieve future success. The second example that shows how demographic changes have introduced changes in the workplace is the way leadership is done. In the past, leadership was all about command and control. Today, it is about engagement. Leaders are expected to engage their followers with the aim of harvesting good ideas which have been found to drive bottom-line outcomes. Another significant change in the workplace is that business used to be done at a local level, now it is global (Engelmeier, 2014).

Technological advancement

Technological advancement has also brought new opportunities and challenges to today's leaders. Of concern is the challenge it has brought to today's leaders. As new technologies emerge, leaders are finding their technological skills becoming obsolete. This prompts them to find means to use the new gadgets for their advantage. In the present scenario, innovation in the technological world seems to be overpowering execution, an aspect that continues to cause nightmare to leaders.

Globalization

Globalization is another factor that has brought changes in the workplace, and in turn, created new challenges to leaders. Of great concern is the diversity. It is apparent that the current global workplace trends have led to the emergence of tensions. As such, today's leaders are experiencing enormous challenges in managing diversity in the global context. Moreover, it is surprising that diversity at the workplace is accompanied by exclusion; thus, creating a critical workplace issue (Mor Barak, 2013). Today's workforce demands fairness and equality in employment, and these new demands cannot be met under the traditional leadership framework.

What Are Ways To Overcome Those Problems?

In principle, new challenges require innovative solutions. This implies that the effectiveness of leadership in organizations will depend on the strategies that leaders will adopt to overcome the emerging challenges. Some of these solutions include inclusive leadership, training of leaders, and collaboration through inclusive workplace model.

Inclusive leadership

Inclusive leadership is deemed ideal for addressing challenges associated to demographic shift. Engelmeier (2014) posits that there are both internal and external benefits of inclusive leadership as a way to counter demographic shifts. He outlines some of the internal benefits as boosting employees' engagement and improved productivity. On the other hand, he cites alignment with markets as a key benefit that drives bottom-line success in organizations. According to Mor Barak (2013) an inclusive workplace model exhibits numerous benefits. It values individual and intergroup differences, cooperates and contributes to the society, collaborates with stakeholders at all levels, and meets the needs of disadvantaged groups. This implies that an inclusive leadership model is ideal for addressing diversity challenges in the workplace.

Training of leaders

Technological advancement is another aspect that has created challenges to today's leaders in the workplace. To address this problem, continuous training for leaders is necessary, in order to ensure that they use technology for their advantage.

What Can Lead To The Success Or Failure Of A Company Due To Good/Bad Leadership?

In retrospect, good leadership is always accompanied by the success of an organization. This implies that supporting leaders, especially by other members within an organization, especially at the senior management level enhances the realization of good leadership benefits. When this occurs, organizational effectiveness in terms of satisfaction, productivity and high quality of products, or services becomes a reality. An outstanding example of organizational success due to good leadership can be provided by the Apple Company. Steve Jobs took the leadership of the company when it was at the verge of collapsing and steered the company to success (Shontell, 2017).

On the other hand, bad leadership has undesirable outcomes. This is attributable to the failures of the leader to uphold the virtues of ethical leadership. An example of company failure due to bad leadership is provided by Enron Company. Exxon Company collapsed as a result of bad leadership that was demonstrated by the lack of accountability, integrity and selfishness. It is reported that leaders used coercive means to manipulate auditors. They also manipulated financial statements to reflect high turnovers, in order to win customers' satisfaction. All these unethical leadership practices led to the collapse of the company that had reported significant progress during the initial stages (Johnson, 2003).

Conclusion

In a brief conclusion, leadership has become essential for the success of today's organizations. This signifies a departure from the past when management was considered as the only tool available for organization's resources utilization. Its popularity is attributable its benefits in organizations, including improvement in production, improved quality of products and services, and increased competitiveness.

However, it is worth noting leadership can bring success or failure in an organization. In practice, good leadership is believed to generate appreciable returns, whereas bad leadership brings failure. Good leaders can be identified through the use of leadership theories which define characteristics of good leaders. Some of the main characteristics of a good leader include ability to motivate, self-confident, attentive, ambitious, and honesty. In contrast, bad leaders are self-centered, coercive, non-empathizers, and non-focused.

15

Despite the need for leadership in today's workplace, leaders are faced with numerous challenges which impair its effectiveness, as well as the success of organizations. Some of these challenges include demographic shifts, globalization and technological advancements. However, new solutions to these challenges are being developed. For instance, inclusive leadership has proven to be effective in addressing diversity; whereas training solves challenges associated to change in technology.

References

Johnson, C. (2003). Enron's Ethical Collapse: Lessons for Leadership Educators. *Journal of Leadership Education, 2*(1), 45-56.

Bertocci, D. I. (2009). *Leadership in Organizations.* Lanham, MD: University Press of America.

Lunenburg, F. C. (2012). Power and Leadership: An Influence Process. *International Journal of Management, Business, and Administration, 15*(1), 1-9.

Stogdill, R. M. (1974). *Handbook of Leadership.* New York, NY: Free Press.

George, J. M., & Gareth, J. (2005). *Understanding and Managing Organizational Behavior (4th ed.).* Upper Saddle River, NJ: Prentice Hall.

Gibson, L., Ivancevich, J., & Donnelly Jr. J. (2000). *Organizations: Behavior, Structure, Processes (10th ed.).* Boston, MA: Irwin McGraw Hill.

Kotter, J. P. (1992). What Do Leaders Really Do? In J. Gabarro (Eds), *Managing People and Organizations* (pp. 102–14). Boston, ma: Harvard Business School Publications.

Kozak, D. C. (1998). *Leadership.* Erie, PA: Gannon University Magazine.

Kirkpatrick, S., & Locke, E. (1991). Leadership: Do Traits Really Matter. *The Executive, 1991,* 48–60.

Cohn, J., & Moran, J. (2011). *Why Are We Bad at Picking Good Leaders? A Better Way to Evaluate Leadership Potential.* Hoboken, NJ: John Wiley & Sons.

Pandey A. (2014). *Traits of Ledership: Ezee Pezee Skills.* New Delhi, India: Skillizen Learning Solutions Pvt. Ltd.

Engelmeier, S. (2014). *Becoming an Inclusive Leader: How to Navigate the 21st Century Global Workforce.* Minneopolis, MN: InclusionINC Media.

Mor Barak, M. (2013). *Managing Diversity: Toward a Globally Inclusive Workplace*. Thousand

    Oaks, CA: Sage.

Pierce, J. A., & Robinson, R. (2007). *Strategic Management* (10th ed.). New York, NY: McGraw

    Hill.

Shontell, A. (2017; August 24). 11 Unusual Ways Steve Jobs Made Apple The World's Most

    Admired Tech Company. *Business Insider*. Retrieved

    http://www.businessinsider.com/11-unusual-ways-steve-jobs-made-apple-the-worlds-

    most-admired-tech-company-2011-8?IR=T

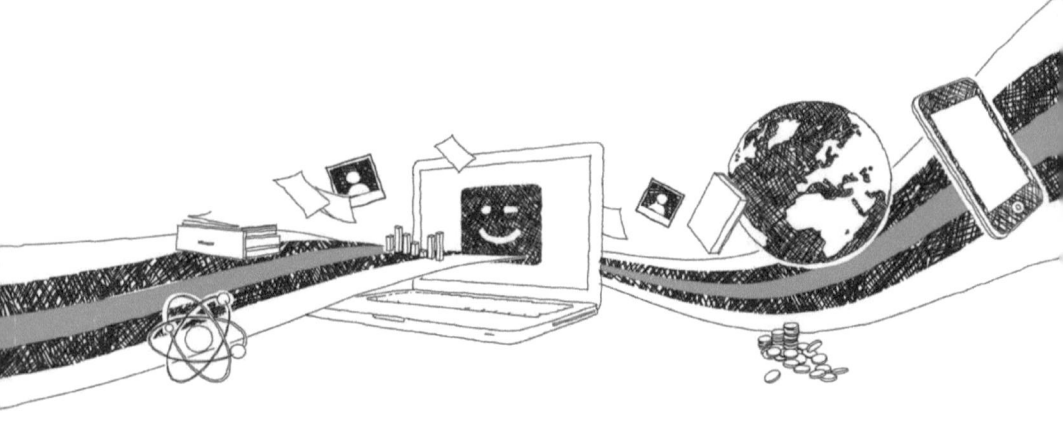
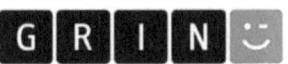